The Virtual Reality Fitness Revolution

A Comprehensive Guide to Workout Routines

Table of Contents

Chapter 1. Introduction

Welcome to a thrilling new frontier in health and fitness! Our Special Report: "The Virtual Reality Fitness Revolution: A Comprehensive Guide to Workout Routines" is designed to be your gateway into an exciting new era where exercise meets the digital world. This is not your typical technical exploration; instead, we invite you to a vibrant journey, packed with engaging information on how to make fitness routines more fun, effective, and thrilling with the power of VR technology. Be ready to discover your new favorite way to stay fit and healthy as we dive into Workout routines like never before. This report will illuminate and captivate, providing a thrilling ride that has the power to completely transform your fitness journey. Don't miss out on revolutionizing your workout routine! The future of fitness is at your fingertips, and inside these pages, the revolution begins.

Chapter 2. Introducing Virtual Reality Fitness

For years, fitness has undergone slow but steady transformations. Introductions of new routines, advanced equipment, and challenging exercises highlight an industry that is continuously evolving. In an era dominated by digital devices, we find the most recent and revolutionary change: Virtual Reality. This technology isn't just for gamers anymore. Instead, it's making a profound impact on the fitness world.

2.1. Understanding Virtual Reality

Virtual reality (VR) can encompass anything in an artificial environment made realistic to the human mind. Viably a convincing simulation, it transports users into a digitally fabricated world thanks to VR headsets. These headsets track and adjust to your movements, rendering 3D images from a slightly different perspective each time, thus creating a surreal immersive experience.

2.2. Bridging the Gap Between Gaming and Fitness

For those who've marveled at the thought of making gaming active or making fitness entertaining, VR is the bridge. VR technology allows users the chance to simultaneously play and stay fit, combining the engaging world of video games with health boosting physical exertion. This combination, it turns out, is an ideal recipe for making workouts much more inviting for everyone.

2.3. The Magic Unveiled: Virtual Reality-Based Fitness

For fitness enthusiasts and casual exercisers alike, engaging and entertaining workouts can sometimes feel like a unicorn. VR Fitness, however, makes that unicorn a reality. As you strap on your VR headset, your living room converts into a virtual gymnasium, a stunning island race track, or even an extraterrestrial battlefield. Your workout routines sprout a new life infused with excitement, completely transforming the way you perceive fitness.

2.4. The Physiology Behind VR Fitness

It's easy to get lost in the enchanting world of VR and forget about an important question: how does it actually maintain or improve physical fitness? Two fundamental components: cardiovascular exercise and muscle toning.

1. Cardiovascular exercise: Most VR games require large and quick body movements, promoting cardiovascular activity. These movements raise your heart rate, effectively turning a gaming session into an aerobic workout.

2. Muscle toning: In VR, you cannot merely press a button to perform an action. Instead, you mimic real-world movements such as throwing, lifting, or jumping. Depending on the intensity of these movements and the duration of gameplay, you can also achieve muscle toning.

2.5. Building A Workout Routine with VR

Building a workout routine using a VR setup involves selecting the correct games and planning a balanced session. Here are some tips to keep in mind:

- Choose a VR game that aligns with your fitness goal. If you're looking for an intense workout, choose a game that requires good cardiovascular activity and prolonged duration.

- Rest is crucial in any fitness routine. It's advisable to start with heavy-duty games, followed by less intensive ones for downtime.

- Having a well-ventilated area with enough space to move around is essential for a smooth, mishap-free VR workout.

- Hydrate and maintain your nutrition intake. Just like any workout, VR fitness demands energy and fluid replenishment.

2.6. Complementing Traditional Workout Routines

While an exciting avenue, VR fitness isn't meant to replace traditional workouts completely. Instead, it supplements and complements your existing routine. VR workouts allow you to burn a few extra calories or maintain your fitness on days when you can't make it to the gym or simply aren't in the mood for traditional workouts. It's a novel and alternative method to keep up the interest and continue your fitness journey seamlessly.

2.7. The Future of Fitness: Advanced VR Offerings

Just as the fitness landscape has evolved, so too will VR Fitness. As VR technology progresses, we'll likely witness introductions of multiplayer games allowing remote workout sessions with friends, integrating wearable tech to track vital health indicators during your VR workout, or offering more specialized training regimes. The possibilities are boundless.

By merging the digital world with physical fitness, VR Fitness offers a novel approach to getting and staying fit. This technology breathes fresh life into your fitness regimen, serving as a testament to innovation's power to revolutionize how we take care of our bodies and minds. Welcome to the new reality of fitness. The virtual expedition has just begun!

Chapter 3. Evolution of Fitness: From Dumbbells to VR Headsets

The journey of fitness, as an integral part of our lifestyle, has witnessed numerous transformations in the methods and modalities of exercise. From the lifting of bulky iron weights to the utilization of machine assistance for targeted workouts, the evolution has been remarkable. However, the advent and integration of virtual reality (VR) into fitness have been a game-changer, quite literally, and on a revolutionary scale.

3.1. The Early Days of Fitness

In the early days of fitness, exercise was more of a necessity rather than a leisure activity. Physical labor was prevalent, and the daily routines of most individuals involved strenuous physical activities. However, the need for purposeful physical exercise rose with the advent of more sedentary lifestyles.

This gave birth to the era of traditional weight training, where fitness enthusiasts would spend endless hours lifting hefty cast-iron dumbbells and barbells. Initially existing as a subculture, resistance training slowly found its place in mainstream society as an effective method of building physical strength and endurance.

3.2. The Equipment Evolution

In the following decades, fitness took a more structured form with the development of equipment made specifically for exercising. Gymnasiums sprung into existence equipped with exercise machines specifically designed to exercise different sets of muscles. Traditional weights were replaced or complemented with these machines to allow for a more targeted and safe approach.

Machines like treadmills, stationary bikes, ellipticals, cable machines, and rowing machines were introduced. The advantage of the gym machines over traditional weights was the minimized risk of injury, regulated intensity, and specificity of muscle group usage.

During this phase, we also saw the initiation of structured workout regimes, gym memberships, personal trainers, and a boom in the fitness industry.

3.3. The Digital Impact

The digital age left its indelible mark on the world of fitness as well. Fitness DVDs and television shows became popular, allowing people to follow along with workout routines at home. This transition marked the commencement of remote fitness, empowering individuals to keep fit without stepping foot in a gym.

Soon after, the internet explosion led to the proliferation of fitness apps, online workout classes, and digital personal trainers. Online fitness programs and applications surged in popularity, offering a wide array of workouts that catered to different fitness levels, goals, and preferences.

3.4. Virtual Reality: Shaping the Future of Fitness

Virtual reality, considered the apex of technological advancement, started making its mark in the fitness world around the mid-2010s. VR fitness programs allow users to experience an immersive workout environment from the comfort of their homes. Its consumer appeal lies in its ability to make fitness fun, combining the exciting elements of video games with intense exercise routines.

VR has introduced a whole new level of interactivity to fitness. With VR headsets, we're able to blend real physical movements with virtual scenarios for a more engaging and immersive experience. VR fitness routines can range from simulated boxing matches to virtual spin classes, enabling users to break a sweat without even realizing they're working out.

3.5. The Pros, Cons, and Future of VR Fitness

There's no denying the immense benefits of VR in fitness: increased engagement, the fun factor, versatile workouts, and convenience are just a few. However, it also poses its own set of challenges such as the need for relatively expensive equipment, suitability issues concerning health and physical abilities of users, and the potential risk of decreased social interaction.

Despite these challenges, the future of VR in fitness appears bright. As the technology advances and becomes more accessible, it is likely to become only more popular among all age groups. Future improvements may even bring more immersive user experiences, improved tracking accuracy, and greater social interactions.

In summary, the fitness journey has been a rollercoaster ride from dumbbells to VR headsets, weaving through various stages of ever-changing methods and modalities of exercise. Today, as VR progressively becomes an integral segment of the fitness industry, we find ourselves on the precipice of the next great leap in how we stay healthy. As technology continues to evolve, fitness routines will continue to become more innovative, engaging, and enjoyable, making us healthier in mind, body, and spirit.

The journey of fitness evolution is far from over. With every advancement in technology, we're getting one step closer to a more integrated, immersive, and exciting way to keep our bodies fit, proving that there's no limit to what we can achieve in the realm of fitness. After all, it would seem fitness is not just a matter of strength and endurance; it's also a matter of creativity and innovation.

Chapter 4. Understanding Virtual Reality: An Insight into the Technology Behind the Screen

Before you embark on this journey to blend fitness with the magic of virtual reality, a brief insight into how VR technology functions is essential. Understanding the technology's intricacies and the method behind the immersion will enable you to entirely fathom the power of your workout routines in the world of VR.

4.1. The Birth of Virtual Reality

The concept of virtual reality is not a twenty-first-century phenomenon. It has been floating around the realm of innovation for longer than you might assume. The first VR head-mounted display, named the "Sword of Damocles", was introduced by Ivan Sutherland and his student Bob Sproull in 1968. Though the technology was cumbersome, the genesis had taken place. Today, we find ourselves immersed in a more user-friendly and advanced form of VR, which has expanded its wings beyond science and has dived deep into entertainment, education, and, of course, fitness.

4.2. The Fundamentals of Virtual Reality

Virtual reality operates on the concept of creating a simulated environment that can be interacted with in a seemingly real or physical way. The environment generated through virtual reality technology is visually immersive, creating a feeling of real-world presence. This immersion is called a 'computer-generated immersive environment'.

The primary goal of VR technology is to create a sensory experience that involves sight, touch, hearing, and at times even smell. The head-mounted display (HMD) has high-density pixel screens and lenses to ensure a wide field of view for the user. This creates a sense of being 'inside' a digital world rather than looking at it from outside.

4.3. The Hardware

VR technology is not confined to a single device. It involves an array of hardware components working in sync to transport you smoothly into a parallel universe. The primary hardware components of a VR setup are:

1. VR Headset: The first and the most visually prominent component of the VR hardware kit is the Headset. It is the primary device responsible for projecting the virtual environment to the user. It consists of high-resolution screens, wide-angle lenses, accelerometers, and gyroscopes.

2. Tracking System: Tracking systems are crucial for VR as they monitor the user's movements and relay them back to the system to reflect them in the virtual environment. These tracking systems could be based on mechanical, ultrasonic, optical, or magnetic technologies. They help in registering even the smallest movements, such as the turn of your head or the flick of your wrist.

3. VR Controllers: VR Controllers, physical devices users hold, provide inputs to the VR environment. They come in various shapes and sizes, from handheld devices like joysticks to wearable glove-based controllers. These devices interpret real-world actions, like grabbing or throwing, into the virtual world.

4. Computers and Processors: Last but not least, the VR hardware

setup requires a high-performing computer. The computer should have a powerful graphics processing unit and processor to support the heavy rendering that VR applications demand.

4.4. Immersion and Presence

For a genuinely transformative VR experience, the user needs to feel genuinely embedded within the digital creation. This encapsulation is possible through two essential components of VR: Immersion and Presence.

Immersion is the measure of how effectively the virtual reality system can create a detailed and convincing sensory environment, while presence refers to the user's subjective psychological response to a VR system. It indicates the extent to which the user feels 'present' in the virtual environment.

4.5. The Software behind VR Workout Experiences

Now that we understand how the hardware works to create an immersive experience, let's take a short stroll through the software behind these magical transformations.

VR software architectures are numerous and varied, but almost all come under two broad categories: game-based engines (like Unity or Unreal) and Web-based platforms (like A-Frame or React 360). These platforms help create the fully interactive, multi-sensorial experiences that make VR fitness apps so engaging.

These software not only render the environment but also take note of the user's position, movements, and interactions to provide real-time feedback. They simulate the laws of physics to make sure the interactions seem as realistic as possible. These software systems thus help to blur the line between imagination and reality.

4.6. The Future of VR Technology in Fitness

Just like how smartphones redefined communication, VR is poised to reshape our exercise routines. By digitizing workouts, VR introduces an engaging and exhilarating component to otherwise repetitive exercises. VR workouts have revolutionized the concept of 'home workouts', allowing people to scale mountains, punch through games, or perform Yoga in serene environments, all while being within the confines of their living room.

The unprecedented times of pandemic lockdowns have further accentuated the acceptance of VR as a serious alternative to traditional gyms. With advancements in machine learning and AI, VR fitness apps are offering personalized routines and real-time feedback, making the workouts more effective and engaging.

To conclude, the cutting-edge technology of Virtual Reality enables us to change our perception of the world and especially our fitness routines. While we are at the brink of broad acceptance of VR in daily fitness regimes, understanding the technology behind the immersion will help us harness its full potential. As we tread forward, we can only imagine the further exciting enhancements VR technology will bring to the fitness universe.

Chapter 5. The Virtual Gym: Exploring the VR Fitness Landscape

The world of fitness has been progressively evolving—from the traditional routine of weightlifting and aerobics to the incorporation of technology via smart wearables. Now, it's time for the next big leap, the integration of Virtual Reality (VR) technology in fitness training. The "Virtual Gym" is an innovative concept that offers an immersive, realistic, and interactive environment for workout routines. This new frontier in fitness promises endless possibilities, transforming monotonous workouts into exciting experiences.

5.1. Emergence of the Virtual Gym

The concept of a "Virtual Gym" emerged from the necessity to incorporate technology into fitness, aiming to make workouts more engaging, enjoyable, and effective. VR technology projects a virtual environment providing a unique workout experience, as it engages both the body and mind during the exercise. Unlike traditional fitness training, where the focus is mostly on physical exertion, a Virtual Gym creates a cognitive connection that can enhance one's motivation and commitment towards fitness.

Imagine a world where your living room can quickly transform into a yoga studio overlooking the dawn-lit mountains. With your VR headset, you can now practice Yoga amid the serenity of a mountain range or even underwater, creating exhilarating experiences that traditional fitness studios can't replicate. This combination of immersive experiences with physical workouts is the essence of a Virtual Gym.

5.2. Hardware and Software Platforms in Virtual Gym

The Virtual Gym's effectiveness depends on its hardware and software. VR Headsets like Oculus Quest, PlayStation VR, HTC Vive, and Valve Index, among others, are widely used for workout routines. Each of these devices offers distinct features and exploration into the virtual world. They house sophisticated sensors that can track your movements and translate them into virtual actions. From the viewpoint of comfort, it is worthwhile investing in a good quality lightweight headset with a high refresh rate and resolution for a smooth VR experience.

The magic is brought alive by VR fitness software applications. Apps like Supernatural, VRWorkout, BoxVR, Holofit, and VZFit offer different genres of workouts. Some focus on aerobic exercises, some on bodyweight exercises, while others dwell on meditation and yoga. Every app is unique, catering to different user preferences from gamified workouts to traditional exercise with a VR twist. Engaging storyline, adaptive difficulty, scoring systems, and global leaderboards are added features that are aimed at making the workouts more enticing while building a community of fitness enthusiasts.

5.3. Training Techniques in Virtual Gym

Virtual Gyms offer a slew of training techniques that are classified into strength workouts, cardio workouts, flexibility routines, and balance exercises.

Strength workouts in VR primarily use bodyweight exercises. By simulating objects and their weights, the applications create resistance against which the user muscles work, generating a similar effect to weightlifting.

Cardio workouts are often gamified and could involve actions akin to boxing or rhythmic catchy beats that you hit or dodge. Not only do you burn calories, but you also improve coordination amid an immersive stimulating experience.

Flexibility routines and balance exercises mostly center around virtual Yoga or Tai Chi classes. These exercises help ease tension, improve posture, and encourage bodily awareness and mindfulness.

Furthermore, data tracking is a standard feature in most apps. User's heart rate, calories burned, movement count, and session duration are commonly tracked metrics providing great insight on workout performance and areas of improvement.

5.4. Overcoming the Challenges

While there is a lot of potential and excitement around the concept of a Virtual Gym, it's also crucial to recognize the potential challenges and roadblocks.

Firstly, there is a cost associated with acquiring a VR setup— the headset, the controllers, and in some cases, additional hardware like PCs or consoles. However, as technology advances and becomes more widespread, these costs are likely to decrease.

Secondly, the physical space required: VR workouts demand a certain amount of space to ensure safety, so users have to manage their surroundings effectively. Solutions for this are being explored, with the advancement of technology like 'Guardian systems' that map the real-world environment to prevent users from bumping into objects.

Lastly, VR workouts are a solitary experience, which some may find isolating. However, the development of social VR fitness classes where users can join live workout sessions with others worldwide makes it possible to bring back the social aspect of fitness.

5.5. The Future of the Virtual Gym

The future of Virtual Gyms is incredibly promising. Picture entering a Virtual Gym and having an AI trainer customizing a program based on your fitness history, preferred workout style, and current mood using advanced analytics. Or participating in global competitions right from your living room. With ongoing research in haptic technology, tactile feedback during workouts would be an exciting feature to look forward to, taking VR workouts to a new level of realism.

In conclusion, Virtual Gyms present an exciting new frontier in fitness, giving everyone an opportunity to overcome geographical barriers, time constraints, or even shyness in public setups. As more people adopt this technology, the Virtual Gym is set to transform the way we perceive fitness, making working out an exciting, immersive, and comprehensive experience, much more than just an obligation or routine. Enjoy the ride into this revolutionary digital world; the future of fitness is here!

Chapter 6. Game-Based Workouts: Breathing Fun into Exercise

Working out can often feel like a chore, particularly when the activities involved are repetitive or lack engagement factor. One of the most invigorating aspects of Virtual Reality fitness is its ability to breathe new life into mundane workout routines, offering an interesting blend of game-based workouts that make exercise enjoyable. By combining physical activity with immersive gaming experiences, VR fitness is truly revolutionizing our approach to personal health.

6.1. The Essence of Game-Based Workouts

Game-based workouts involve incorporating elements of video games – such as challenges, rewards, and fun narratives – into fitness routines. As you progress in these 'fitness games', you naturally accomplish exercise goals along the way. Imagine playing a sword fighting game; as you swashbuckle your way through, you're simultaneously working out your arms, shoulders, and core. Game-based workouts veil the strain of traditional exercise behind an immersive interactive veil, making the pursuit of fitness a pleasurable activity rather than a demanding task.

VR technology takes the essence of game-based workouts to a new level. It immerses you into a virtual playground where fitness goals intertwine with game objectives, engaging you not just physically but also mentally and emotionally. These game-based experiences are meticulously designed to incite your motivation, enhance your effort, and ensure your commitment to your fitness journey.

6.2. The Evolution of Game-Based Workouts

The concept of game-based workouts is not entirely novel. From the basic rhythm games of old to the more modern kinetic games — recall the Wii Fit or Kinect Adventures — digital interactive workouts have been subtly evolving. However, with VR technology redefining gaming experiences, the conception of game-based workouts has taken a quantum leap forward, singlehandedly catapulting users into a realm where the border between gaming and workout melds into a hazy mist.

VR fitness games often combine different exercise types, seamlessly integrated to keep the gameplay lively and varied. Some games incorporate high-intensity interval training, while others might feature activities like boxing, dancing, or even archery. Each category of games tax and hone different sets of muscles and provide diverse intensity levels to cater to all fitness levels and preferences.

6.3. Popular Game-Based VR Workouts

The market brims with various VR fitness games aimed at diverse fitness goals and gaming tastes. A few note-worthy ones are:

- Beat Saber: A rhythm-based game where you slice beats (or blocks) with a light saber. Your ducking, strafing, and slashing motions are equivalent to a heart-thumbing cardio workout.

- BoxVR: BoxVR makes you feel like a boxing champion by throwing punches to the rhythm of high-energy music. It's a fantastically engaging way to experience high-impact cardio.

- Creed: Rise to Glory: Train with the legendary Rocky Balboa and step into the ring to become a boxing champ, while physically living every punch, dodge, and uppercut.

- OhShape: A combination of fun physical puzzles, dancing, and intense cardio, it has you moving your body in all imaginable angles to match the silhouettes on screen.

Each of these games has its unique approach towards fitness. They leverage the immersive nature of VR to ensure users gradually push their boundaries without even realizing it.

6.4. Customizing Game-Based Workouts

While VR games bring fun into workouts, that's only half the story. Their real success lies in their ability to be molded to individual preferences and requirements. Some games let you customize the level of intensity, the genre of music, or the type of movements, often resulting in workouts tailored to your specific needs.

The level of exertion in VR workouts can be tuned to throw challenges that gradually improve your fitness over time. This flexibility improves the remaining lifespan of these games – the better you get, the game recalibrates to your new normal, maintaining the right balance of challenge and engagement needed for sustained physical development.

6.5. Conclusion: The Future of Game-Based Workouts

The evolution of game-based workouts in VR signals an exciting future for fitness. Turning workouts into immersive game experiences complements diverse fitness goals and undeniably enhances individual motivation. Game-based VR workouts are more than sheer amusement, they provide an unconventional pathway that shifts fitness from a daunting obligation to an enticing playtime.

VR takes game-based workouts from something you have to do towards something you want to pursue. As technology advances and more creative minds explore this genre, the line separating games from workouts will blur even further, creating engaging fitness-play hybrids that promise engaging and effective fitness solutions.

Glimpsing into the horizon of this potential-filled future, we see gaming and wellness joining hands to pioneer a fitness revolution like never before. The only questions that remain are: How will you choose to indulge in this revolution? Which game workout will be your next playtime?

Chapter 7. Tailoring Your VR Workout: A Guide to Personalisation

With the emergence of Virtual Reality (VR) technology, fitness routines can now be tailored and personalised to encapsulate everything from your fitness level, interests, and goals to your physical surroundings. This evolution in exercise approaches provides the unique opportunity to blend the allure of digital interaction with the tangible benefits of physical movement. Let's explore this in-depth, and learn to tailor your VR workouts.

7.1. Assessing Your Fitness Level

Before diving headfirst into any fitness routine, it's important to determine your base fitness level. This applies equally to VR exercise. Health attributes you should consider include cardiorespiratory fitness, muscular strength and endurance, flexibility, and body composition.

VR fitness platforms typically offer benchmark tests that help you gauge where you are at the start of your fitness journey and provide an accurate reference point for personal goal setting. Pay heed to these evaluations as they serve as the foundation of your tailored VR program.

7.2. Understanding Your Goals

Establishing clear, defined fitness goals at the outset is essential for success. Whether you want to lose weight, gain muscle, increase stamina, boost flexibility, or simply increase your daily activity, your VR fitness routine can be customized to meet these objectives.

Set SMART (Specific, Measurable, Achievable, Relevant, Time-bound) goals. Make these targets a combination of short-term and long-term goals. Your short-term goals will serve as stepping stones to your long-term goals, and every milestone reached fuels you with motivation.

7.3. Choosing Your VR Exercise Environment

An advantage of VR fitness is being able to immerse yourself in any locale imaginable. From the tranquility of a deserted beach to the energetic applause in a packed stadium, your VR workout can transport you anywhere.

Selection of environments often depends on the type of activity and personal tastes. Yoga enthusiasts might prefer peaceful, natural vistas while those running a marathon might prefer a cityscape. Don't underestimate the power of virtual environments; they can greatly influence your motivation and commitment.

7.4. Selecting Appropriate Fitness Games and Programs

After understanding your fitness level and goals, and deciding on your preferred environments, you need to choose the right VR games and programs. There's a vast array of fitness games and programs available, each providing unique experiences and catering to different fitness goals.

Cardio-focused individuals can explore games that involve a lot of movement. Strength-trainers might play games where virtual weights are employed. Balance and flexibility enthusiasts could participate in games involving dance or yoga. Do your research and find what suits you best.

7.5. Incorporating Non-VR Training

6While VR training offers a fascinatingly immersive experience, incorporating non-VR exercises into your routine is beneficial. Traditional exercises like weightlifting, cycling, running, and bodyweight exercises provide specific benefits and incorporating these into your VR routine can make for a well-rounded fitness program.

7.6. Monitoring Progress

Finally, consistent tracking and monitoring of your progress is vital. Many VR fitness platforms provide in-platform trackers which record various metrics including calories burned, time spent exercising, and performance in games or modules. Regularly checking in on these and reassessing goals when necessary ensures continuous improvement and helps maintain motivation.

Virtual Reality has shattered the limits of traditional fitness routines, allowing for personalised, immersive experiences that make fitness engaging and fun. Whether you're a fitness enthusiast or just starting, VR fitness has something for everyone: it's truly a revolution in personal health and wellbeing. By tailoring your VR workout, you harness the heightened effectiveness and enjoyment this emerging technology brings. Remember to be patient with the process, savor the journey, and above all else, enjoy your workout. The future of fitness is here.

Chapter 8. Benefits and Concerns: Understanding the Pros and Cons of VR Fitness

As much as virtual reality has opened up unique opportunities for fitness enthusiasts globally, it comes with its share of merits and drawbacks. In this section, we explore the pros and cons of VR fitness, providing invaluable insights to assist you in making informed decisions.

8.1. Benefits of VR Fitness

Although countless benefits come with VR Fitness, we will focus on the most significant ones; Increased Motivation, Accessibility, Variety, Data Tracking, and Immersive Experience.

Increased Motivation

The most prominent advantage of VR fitness is probably the increased motivation that users experience. VR technology replaces the monotony of a routine workout with an engaging and exciting virtual environment. Participants can climb mountains, explore mythical worlds, dance with virtual partners, or play high octane games - all while burning calories. The level of engagement in VR fitness makes workouts fly by, hence motivating users to exercise for longer periods.

Accessibility

Generally, VR fitness offers accessibility like never before. Users are no longer confined to gym hours or classes; they can now work out in the comfort of their homes at any time, as long as they have VR equipment. Moreover, since travel time is eliminated, users can fit in a quick workout when they have spare moments, making it an excellent solution for individuals with busy schedules.

Variety

One of the main reasons people become disillusioned with fitness is the lack of variety. VR training provides a solution to this problem. There are hundreds of virtual reality fitness games and applications available, spanning various activities like boxing, dancing, climbing, yoga, and more. This wide range of options ensures that workouts never become monotonous.

Data Tracking

With VR Fitness, all your data like heart rate, calorie count, time spent exercising, and your performance stats can be tracked and saved. This valuable data can help users stay motivated, assess their progress, and decide what parameters they need to work on.

Immersive Experience

VR offers a level of immersion that traditional workouts can't match. It allows users to escape reality and immerse themselves in a completely different world, making workouts enjoyable and exciting. The immersive nature of VR fitness can make users forget they're exercising, which could lead to longer workout sessions without feeling laborious.

8.2. Concerns about VR Fitness

Like anything else, VR fitness, too, comes with certain downsides. The common concerns include Initial Investment, Motion Sickness, Safety Concerns, Lack of Social Interaction, and Future Dependency.

Initial Investment

The major barrier to VR fitness for many is the high initial cost. VR headsets and compatible hardware can be expensive. While the prices are gradually decreasing with technological advances and increased manufacturing, these costs can be limiting for some users.

Motion Sickness

VR-induced motion sickness, also known as "cybersickness," is a common problem for some VR users. Symptoms can include dizziness, nausea, disorientation, and sometimes even oculomotor problems such as eye strain and headaches. Not everyone will experience these, and many can adapt over time, but it's worth being aware of the possibility.

Safety Concerns

While exercising in VR, users can sometimes forget about the real-world space around them. This neglect can result in injuries from tripping over objects, running into walls, or overextending one's boundaries. Therefore, a safe play area free of any obstacles is a must when using VR for fitness.

Lack of Social Interaction

Although some VR Fitness apps offer online multiplayer modes, they still can't replicate the motivational camaraderie found in a class or gym setting. Face-to-face social interaction during workouts is missing, which could be a drawback for those who thrive in such environments.

Future Dependency

Dependency on VR for fitness can be a concern too. Exercise should be about improving one's health and wellness, but the addictive nature of the VR gaming experience could turn this essential health activity into a gaming dependency.

In conclusion, despite the compelling benefits, the drawbacks of VR fitness can't be ignored. The decision to adopt this technology should depend on personal preferences, needs, and health considerations. As the field continues to grow and evolve, we can look forward to solutions that minimize these drawbacks and maximize the benefits, transforming the fitness landscape.

Chapter 9. Staying Motivated with VR: Gamification and Beyond

Virtual reality (VR) has transformed countless industries, and fitness is no exception. Leveraging powerful tools such as gamification, this emerging technology has the potential to supercharge motivation and reinvent the exercise experience.

9.1. Gamification: Turning Workouts into a Game

An integral part of VR fitness is the use of gamification—the application of game design elements in non-gaming settings. In this case, a workout environment. It's no secret that games are designed to be addictive, with quests, rewards, and social dynamics that keep you coming back day after day. VR fitness uses these mechanics to fuel motivation and make workouts feel less like a chore, and more like an entertaining activity.

To understand how gamification enhances workouts, consider how many people abandon traditional exercise routines. Strenuous workouts are often difficult to adhere to due to lack of immediate, observable results. Gamification, with immediate rewards in the form of points, levels, or completed challenges, offers that needed encouragement.

Some VR fitness programs employ the use of leaderboards to spark a sense of competition among users. By working to outperform others, you're likely to push yourself harder than if you were exercising just for personal gains. This subtle competition leverages our innate desire to win, driving us to stick with our routines and continually strive to improve.

Another important aspect within VR gamification is the personalized rewards system. Virtual rewards—like new game levels, avatars, or virtual equipment—to celebrate progress are terrific motivators. These perks can be tied to personal milestones, such as beating your best time or completing a certain number of workouts, making each exercise session feel productive and fulfilling.

9.2. The Role of Immersion in Motivation

Beyond gamification, VR offers a unique sense of presence and immersion that is difficult to replicate in non-VR workouts. This quality contributes to motivation by providing a captivating and engaging workout atmosphere. You're not just running on a treadmill; you could be sprinting away from zombies, or racing through a lush fantasy world.

This form of escapism simultaneously provides distractions from the physical discomfort associated with exercise and contributes to the sustained motivation for Physical Exercise (PE). As your mind becomes engrossed in the VR world, you effectively forget about the arduous nature of your workout, enabling you to exercise longer and with greater intensity.

Moreover, the immersive quality of VR directly counteracts one of the common obstacles in maintaining regular exercise-regiment boredom. With VR, no two workouts need to be the same. You can change environments, difficulty levels, and even the type of exercise you're doing, creating a variety-filled workout regimen.

Further enhancing immersion, most VR fitness apps feature atmospheric audio and haptic feedback. The surround-sound audio immerses you in the workout, while haptic feedback provides a physical response—like feeling the vibration of a punch landed—which adds a deeper level of interactivity and presence.

9.3. Combining Physical and Virtual: The Intersection of Two Realities

VR Fitness bridges the gap between physical exertion and digital entertainment. Advanced motion tracking technology allows your physical movements to translate into corresponding actions within the game. Punching, ducking, jumping, and jogging can control your character, enemies, or the environment itself.

This embodiment within the virtual world elevates the exercise experience to more than just calorie burning or muscle building—it transforms it into an embodied narrative. You're not merely a spectator in a digital game; you're an active participant. This active physical engagement not only enhances the fun factor but also contributes to exercise adherence.

9.4. Community Building

Community creation is another crucial component in VR fitness. Many platforms facilitate connections with other users around the world. People can form workout groups, participate in group classes, or even compete in challenges together.

This kind of cooperative or competitive virtual team-mate dynamic adds a layer of sociability that many traditional fitness routines lack. You can share successes, encourage each other toward fitness goals, and form bonds around a shared effort. This sense of belonging can greatly increase exercise persistence and consistency.

9.5. The Future is Now

In conclusion, the combination of gamification, immersion, community involvement, physical-virtual integration, and the sheer entertainment value of VR makes it a strong tool for enhancing exercise motivation. The future of fitness is not years away; it's already here, transforming traditional workouts into immersive, rewarding experiences.

This paradigm shift is only the beginning. With rapid technological advancements, we can anticipate even greater developments in VR fitness. Potential expansions could include incredibly realistic graphics, new fitness modules, or even real-time coaching powered by AI.

So, as we continue to merge the physical with the digital, the future of VR fitness awaits, promising countless ways to inject fun, motivation, and effectiveness into our fitness routines.

Chapter 10. Success Stories: Personal Journeys using VR Fitness

In the realm of health and fitness, as virtual reality evolves by leaps and bounds, countless individuals are discovering its transformative power. Each encounter with VR fitness is a unique tale of transformation and extraordinary results, demonstrating just how big a difference this technological innovation can make. Let's delve into their experiences!

10.1. The Story of John: From Couch Potato to VR Athlete

John was a self-proclaimed 'couch potato,' who exerted more strength in typing away at his computer keyboard than anything else. Going out for a run, doing a set of sit-ups, or even lifting dumbbells sounded almost alien to him. That was, until he stumbled upon VR fitness.

Encouraged by the blend of gaming and exercise, he bought his first VR headset. The first thing he noticed was how immersive the environment was. There was a virtual gym where an animated trainer was doing warm-up stretches. He followed the routine. The experience was surreal, and for the first time, he enjoyed exercising.

As days passed, he realized he was not breathless anymore after climbing one flight of stairs. He was actually getting healthier without even realizing it. VR fitness turned his life around.

10.2. Emily's Experience: VR Combat Fitness

For 30-year-old Emily, who leads a busy lifestyle balancing work and family, going to a gym had fallen by the wayside. Chancing upon an ad for a VR game, she decided to give it a try owing to her love for video games.

She began using a VR fitness game named BoxVR, wherein she was to hit targets following the rhythm of music. It was a world that made her forget she was working out. Before she realized it, she was hooked onto VR fitness.

Within weeks she began to notice her weight shedding, her stamina increasing, and a newfound strength in her arms. No longer was fitness something that had to be squeezed into her schedule; instead, it became a part of her daily routine that she eagerly looked forward to.

10.3. Alex's Escapade: VR Adventures and Dance Fitness

A stay-at-home dad, Alex loved exploring the outdoors. However, children and domestic commitments meant he had to stay indoors more often. VR was his portal back into that world of adventure once again.

Alex decided to embark on an adventure with fitness-based games like "The Thrill of the Fight," a boxing game, and "Creed: Rise to Glory." Much to his surprise, he saw pounds melting away. He then delved into dance fitness with games like "Beat Saber" where he had to slice beats of music with lightsabers, combining his love for Star Wars and dance.

His fitness levels began to skyrocket. VR brought back the joy he used to get from exploring and staying active outdoors, right into his living room.

10.4. Kim's Journey: Overcoming Physical Limitations with the Power of VR

Kim had always believed in living an active lifestyle. But a serious knee injury, followed by surgery, inhibited her from performing strenuous workouts. As days turned into weeks, she couldn't help but miss the feeling of sweat trickling down her forehead after an intense workout.

One fine day, she was introduced to a VR fitness module tailored for people with physical limitations just like her. She took up low-impact exercises, which prevented undue stress on her injured knee, using games like "VZ Fit" which had an array of seated exercises that she could perform using a stationary bike.

VR allowed her to take control of her fitness again without physically hurting herself. Weeks into her new regime, she felt her strength returning, thanks to the power of VR.

10.5. Jake's Transformation: Breaking the Boundaries of Traditional Fitness

Jake, an avid gym-goer, started feeling his routine monotonous after five years of straight weightlifting and treadmill cardio. He needed something innovative to reignite his love for fitness, and VR provided just that.

With games like "Pistol Whip" and "Ring Fit Adventure," he found a new way of working out that was not only fun but also wildly gratifying. He could feel his body getting a full workout, and his endurance levels rose surprisingly. Seeing his physical changes, his peers at the gym were intrigued and soon followed suit.

Virtual reality fitness encapsulated the creativity and fun factor that traditional fitness was generally perceived as lacking. For Jake, and many others, the inclusion of VR in their fitness journey proved to be transformative.

The beauty of VR fitness is that its potential is limitless, matching each person's unique fitness journey with immersive experiences that tread beyond the physical bounds. The health transformations from the formerly sedentary to the fitness-hungry prove that the future of fitness indeed lies within the realm of VR, enhancing personal journeys towards a healthier lifestyle.

These profound personal experiences should be an eye-opener for fitness enthusiasts and novices alike and an encouragement to embrace the exciting opportunities offered by VR. Let the stories of John, Emily, Alex, Kim, and Jake inspire you to embark on your own fitness journey like no other, with the world of virtual reality as your guide and workout partner.

Chapter 11. The Future of VR Fitness: Trends and Predictions

Immersive experiences and beyond is a promise of the virtual reality (VR) technology, extending its reach into various sectors. Health and fitness are increasingly embracing VR to transform traditional workouts into engaging, efficient, and fun activities. Current trends reveal interesting developments on the horizon that are creating a profound shift in the fitness landscape. This chapter explores what we can expect in the future: ranging from highly immersive environments, tailored personal trainers, multiplayer fitness experiences, advancement in haptic feedback, and potential impacts of AI in VR fitness.

11.1. The Rise of Immersive Environments

Physical workouts can sometimes be monotonous, discouraging users from maintaining their fitness routine. VR steps in with a solution: by creating immersive environments that evoke a sense of presence, working out becomes an adventure. Future advancements might include unlimited landscapes to explore and dynamic surroundings that would react to user's movements. Imagine climbing up a mountain, diving under the sea, or floating in space while accomplishing your fitness objectives. The immersive feature combined with the interactive gaming aspect could likely be a gamechanger in keeping users motivated and engaged in their workout sessions.

11.2. Personal Trainers in VR

Already, we see the emergence of AI-controlled personal trainers in VR fitness software. Enabled by a combination of machine learning and biometric data, these virtual coaches are graduating from just simple guiding figures to advanced entities capable of personalizing workouts and providing detailed analysis and feedback. With continual advancements, we expect a future where your virtual coach would understand your stamina, your strengths and weaknesses, schedule, dietary requirement, emotional state, and align the workout plan accordingly. This level of personalization would mark a significant shift from general workout patterns to specific fitness schedules designed for each individual.

11.3. Social Elements and Multiplayer Experiences

One surprising element of VR workouts is their inherent social aspect. Current trends hint towards multiplayer experiences becoming a part of VR fitness. Imagine competing with friends across continents, challenging a random player for a quick match, collaborating on a joint fitness goal, or just sharing the rope in a virtual environment. These interactions add a community aspect into VR fitness. You would be able to share your achievements, get motivation from peers, or exchange tips on exercise techniques, thereby transforming the solitary workout routine into a shared experience.

11.4. Advanced Haptic Feedback

The sense of touch plays a significant role in our interactions with the physical world. Current VR systems primarily rely on visual and audio effects. However, the future holds potential for the tactile sensation to be introduced in our VR workouts, thanks to haptic feedback technology. We could foresee development of haptic suits or gloves that would simulate different textures, resistances, temperature, and impacts. This technology could add another layer of realistic experiences to VR fitness, enhancing the workout effectiveness and reinforcing the sense of presence in the virtual environment.

11.5. AI-Driven Customization and Progress Tracking

AI holds the key to unlock new dimensions in VR fitness. It is likely that the customary fitness metrics would be enriched with real-time data analysis and predictive models. This means your virtual coach would not only guide you during the workout but also anticipate potential injuries based on your form, or suggest meal plans as per your worked up appetite. The progress tracking would be more intuitive involving emotional, mental, and environmental factors apart from the physical ones. This holistic approach could change the way we perceive fitness, broadening its scope beyond muscle building or weight loss, and encompassing overall well-being.

In conclusion, the future of VR fitness offers a landscape teeming with possibilities and breakthroughs that could revolutionize conventional workouts. Blending sophisticated technology, innovative interfaces, and elements of social connection promises to deliver an unprecedented user experience. While these predictions will take time to become widespread, the initial strides towards them are already seen in the fitness tech market. As developers and enthusiasts continue to push boundaries, one thing's for certain — the VR fitness revolution is well underway and its future looks bright and brimming with potential.